Yoga and Spiritual growth

Yoga and Spiritual growth

✦

An explanation of yoga philosophy and lifestyle.

Yogi Yagnesh ShantiOm

iUniverse, Inc.

New York Lincoln Shanghai

Yoga and Spiritual growth
An explanation of yoga philosophy and lifestyle.

iUniverse books may be ordered through booksellers or by contacting:

iUniverse
2021 Pine Lake Road, Suite 100
Lincoln, NE 68512
www.iuniverse.com
1-800-Authors (1-800-288-4677)

ISBN: 978-0-595-47854-5

Printed in the United States of America

Contents

Acknowledgements

Salutations to the inner guru who brings unlimited knowledge and absolute bliss. This book is dedicated to all those who seek the truth and the spiritual way of life. My gratitude goes to my gurus, some whom I have met in the physical form and the ascended masters, who have guided me from the higher realm. May the divine inspiration descend upon you who hold this book in your hand.

Prelude

The origins of the sacred science of yoga is lost in the corridors of time. It was first taught by Lord Shiva who explained it to matsyandranath, and passed down throughout the ages in the form of poetic expositions which were memorized by those who received it. This sacred knowledge was eventually written down in Sanskrit language about five thousand years ago. Many scholars have studied this language in order to gain insight to the sacred science of yoga.

There are many books on the subject of yoga. Some explain the famous postures and exercise of yoga, and some like this book explain the philosophy of yoga. These books are a translation of the original texts which may contain commentaries and or heavily intellectualized which is to my opinion the wrong approach to explaining spiritual concepts. It is not my intention to produce another such book. My intention is to explain the yoga philosophy in a simple language and use my personal experiences to shed light on the spiritual concepts. This book is written in a very simple language and it aims at the modern practitioner. I tried to lay them out for you so you can examine them and gain insight to the deeper meaning on your own.

In the first chapter I have explained and interpreted some famous passages from the old and new testaments, only because the western reader is more familiar with those concepts. By explaining those passages I have made it easier for the reader to grasp the spiritual concepts explained in yoga philosophy. I hope that my personal experiences and interpretations can add some valuable guidance to better understand and practice the principals explained in this book. The words you see in the *italic* format are actual terms used in yoga and are explained in the back of the book under "Terminology"; all terms are listed in alphabetic order.

Keep this book handy as a companion wherever you go and refer to it as a means of inspiration. I hope that you find answers to the mysteries of the universe through your practices.

CHAPTER ONE

Introduction

Yoga! This word means joining or union. Some people believe it to be a form of exercise, which at the best will align or connect the mind and body. In the Classic text of yoga, whose origins go beyond five thousand years, the joining or union is between the individual soul, and the supreme—being or God. The "exercise" of yoga helps in keeping the body healthy. The body is the temple of the soul and spiritual growth is not possible if the body or the mind is in turmoil. Yoga practices which includes exercises, breathing techniques and most importantly meditation, helps us heal physically, mentally, and emotionally so that we are prepared to "experience" our true essence, which is the immortal soul.

The ancient sages were marveling at questions such as, who am I? Why am I here? And what happens when I die? The answers were revealed to them in deep meditation. These ancient yogis were the first humans to come up with the concept of the soul, the true essence within, or the true self. And yoga, also known as the science of self—realization, is a discipline that helps you experience that true self.

This book is about spiritual growth, which means we shall discuss the realm of the spirit. The spirit is intangible and can only be "experienced". It's important to know that Yoga is not a mere philosophy or an act of intellectualization, but a scientific method to help you experience the spiritual. It is scientific because it begins with what is tangible and shows specific methods by which one can connect to the intangible realm of the spirit. According to yoga, the soul is experiencing the limitation of physical universe. After the death of the physical body, the soul is born into the next dimension of existence and will continue on by dying of that level and being born into the next dimension of being and continues its progress until it reaches the most exalted level of existence where there is no duality, and the soul has recognized its true essence to be one with all of creation which is an extension of the all creative force that is God. In this unitive state the creator and created are essentially one. Ancient mystics, and yogis who practiced yoga and meditation over six thousand years ago were perhaps the first people to speak of the existence of the soul, which will continue its journey after death and progresses through several other dimensions of existence until it finally reaches the exalted station of realizing it's true Self. Yogis believe and have proven that one can reach that level right here in this very lifetime, and devised precise techniques to achieve such heightened states of consciousness. For one who has truly experienced such levels of enlightenment nothing is impossible. The mystics and saints have demonstrated such feats as walking on water, levitating, appearing and disappearing and other super natural activity to actually prove that they truly have experienced and live the unitive state in which the creation and the creator are merged. "The father and I are one" is the kind of statement you hear from a genuine yogi, one who has achieved the unitive state.

In essence there is no duality and all existence at every level is an emanation of the divine creative force. Realization of this truth is the actual experience of it or yoga.

Never should the reader approach ideas expressed in this book for intellectual debate. Spiritual truth should become one's personal experience, and Yoga is the discipline used to reach that experience. It is often difficult to describe such intense spiritual experiences, and words become inadequate, yet the yearning to share these experiences and findings with the rest of humanity has been the driving force behind the scriptures, explaining the experience and the discipline.

The teachings have been passed down from the teacher who acted as an experienced guide, to the student who would in turn experience the truth. Both the mystical utterances received in deep meditation, and the actual discipline used to reach those experiences were memorized as poetic passages and eventually written down.

Although the teachings are timeless and have survived the dark corridors of time, the actual text is only a few thousand years old.

The goal of this book is to explain the discipline required to reach these spiritual experiences, we hope that the reader will have a clear understanding of the process, and the how or why of it; but to gain the experience one must put the teachings into daily practice. It is rare to find a living guide, who will lead you according to your unique individuality. The true teacher has had the experience and is both able and willing to take your hand and help you along the way; not intellectually but from his own experience. Not all who achieve the experience choose to teach it.

First, one has to recognize the truth, which may seem like intellectualization, then comes the realization of that truth which is intuitive; not just by faith, but from the actual experience which is beyond description, and it goes beyond reason and even faith. Once the experience is achieved, the practitioner will want to re-live the experience and with more discipline, is able to reach that level of consciousness again and again until he or she gains enough experience to be able to guide others to the summit, but not everyone is qualified or is willing enough to teach others. This book will give the foundation and most necessary information to put you on the path, and let you develop your own experiences along the way. Keep this book as your companion along the path of spiritual growth.

When we speak of a third person we may refer to that person as he, this is due to the limitations of the English language and is not intended to be about gender superiority, specially when we speak of the divine. Since the divine manifests in all forms and yet is exalted above gender, but our limited minds will express it as male or female, God or Goddess. The main requirement in the spiritual path is open-mindedness, please don't limit yourself with pre-conceptions and open your heart and mind to delve deep into the realm of the spirit. This book is not for fast readers. It's full of profound spiritual truths, so I recommend that you read each paragraph carefully and contemplate on its content so that you may grasp it's deeper meaning. May the divine teacher guide you to the mysteries of the spiritual.

Genesis of the Manifest Universe

"In the beginning there was God, and the word was with God, and the word was God".

This passage is perhaps the most important information revealed to humanity. Yogis have spoken of this truth for millennia. Contemplation on this passage opens new insight and gives us inspiration in the path of spiritual growth.

"… In the beginning," When is the beginning?

Time is a by-product of the three dimensional universe. The three dimensions are length, width, and height. The time factor comes in when traveling from one point to another within the three-dimensional space, because this would require the passage of time. So the time factor is a by-product of the manifested universe. Before the creation of the manifest universe, time didn't exist and the phrase "in the beginning" really means at a time before time, which is beyond our understanding. This is why they say the divine creator has always been and shall exist forever.

"… And the word was with God," A word represents an idea. When I say, "book", in your mind you visualize a bunch of pages of paper bound together with covers to protect it. When I say, "table" in your mind you see a round, square or rectangular surface supported by four legs. So the "word" is an idea that exists in the mind. As the word came forth from God the idea of the creation was released into existence. But pay attention to where it said "… and the word was God". God is the idea of creation. So the idea of creation, the creation itself and God are one and the same. Please read the passage again and contemplate on it.

We also heard people say, "God created everything out of nothing". There can't be "nothing" if there was God. So what really happened is not just the universe and time but all the infinite spiritual dimensions came into existence out of the divine will. Therefore just like the rays of sun the manifest universe is emanating out of the divine. Although the rays of the sun are not the sun itself, yet it is because of the sun that there is light. So because God is, that everything exists. So at a deeper level of consciousness you can say that the creation and the creator are one. This is a mystical truth that can only be realized in deep meditation, not through intellectual debate.

Mankind as a physical being, with a limited mind cannot fathom the station of the Creator. As much as an ant cannot understand a human being, man can never fully "Understand" the supreme divinity or God. The divine creator is the purest and highest level of existence.

Somewhere else it is written, "God created man in his own image". Now we all know God is not a physical being. This verifies that humanity is of the spirit, a spiritual being, and essentially divine. It is because of the soul within us that we inquire into the deep secrets of life and death, or feel a yearning for a deeper connection or higher purpose. When we look up at the starry night we ask then who created all this? This is unique in human beings and animals never reach this state of spiritual wonderment. Therefore since man is "made in the image of his creator"—meaning he is a spiritual being—he is capable of experiencing the mystical state of union with God. This is accomplished through the process of yoga, which we will discuss in detail in the following chapters. But first we need to discuss another important mystical truth.

Adam, Eve & the Garden of Eden

Let's contemplate on the story of Adam and Eve to gain more insight on this subject.

In one aspect, Adam and Eve are really one and the same. They represent the logical and the emotional facet of human species. But to reduce confusion let's approach them as separate entities. It is said that Adam and Eve were angels created in God's image. Meaning that they are spiritual beings that came forth from the divine, and were roaming in the Garden of Eden. This place (the garden of Eden) represents the exalted and blissful state of unity with the divine, and all of creation.

"But they (Adam & Eve) ate of the forbidden fruit." This forbidden fruit represents selfish ego. God gave man the freedom to choose, and warned him of the destructive effects of egotism. Yet man chose to taste this fruit, longing to gain an "identity", and suddenly he was separated from God, removed from the bliss of oneness with his creator and was brought down to earth (Physical existence), where he is experiencing the phenomenal universe, which is governed by natural laws. He is lost in a dream world of limitations, forgetting that he is truly an image of the creator, who is limitless, infinite and immortal. It is important to note that transcending that selfish ego is the only way back to our true-self.

Yoga shows us the way back to our true-self, our birth right as God's children roaming in the blissful state of nearness to the divine.

The yogi at the final stages of his or her quest is said to have achieved *samadhi*, ecstasy or *nirvana*. This stage is experienced in deep meditation. With continuous practice the yogi can remain in this state constantly. This level of consciousness may not be achieved in a short period of time except by the will of God. In fact it may take several lifetimes to achieve this. But it is the journey that is important. The dedicated yogi gains new and exciting experiences along the path and this makes the journey very pleasant and interesting.

Patience, dedication, and humility are most necessary for this path. Reading inspirational books, attending *satsang*, being close to a living master or guru and to practice with a group from time to time keeps you excited about what you are trying to achieve. There are no shortcuts and there is no compromising. The lower self must die for the higher self to shine forth, this is truly being "reborn"; which is a concept that has been known to the yogis for thousands of years. Traditionally once an aspirant chooses to follow the path of yoga, he will die of his old identity and is given a new name which may change again and again as he achieves higher levels of achievement.

In fact traditionally yogis and sages have left the conventional life, renounced family, friends and all of their belongings and went to the forest and caves of the Himalayas to gain spiritual merits. This is often considered the extreme and many modern Yogis continue with family life and their function in society. The key is to be a renounced at heart. Knowing that everything in this life is temporary and no happiness comes from acquisition of materials, which eventually decay and perish, the true yogi lives "in the world" but is not "of the world". So complete detachment from the world, avoidance of big money and fortune are the sure signs of a genuine yogi. The true masters never refer to themselves as master and practice much humility and are engaged in the service of the world. It should be fully understood that all spiritual merits come only to those who truly have transcended their lower nature and particularly the ego-self. The true self is not the name we are known as, not the occupation we are engaged in or the gender we know ourselves to be, the true-self transcends name, gender, occupation, nationality, race and everything else that we identify ourselves with. This may seem extreme or impossible to grasp, but little by little as we get to know the true self through the practice, we let go of the ego.

Child of God

Look at a newborn baby. This is an innocent being. He knows no fear, no hatred, no jealousy, or greed. Cannot fathom the violent act of killing nor is he even aware of his own physical body, does not know if he requires food or water. This is an innocent child.

This very same baby after eventually opening his eyes will begin developing the ego-mind. It is important to understand the ego mind. The ego mind has entangled the soul in maya or illusion. Here is how we develop the ego-mind. Our senses (*Indrias*) provide information about the environment, the mind gathers this data, and the intellect (Bodhi) begins to analyze the information and gives rise to ego (*Ahamkara*). I don't mean selfish ego, at least not at the very beginning of such development. The ego is the separation of all that is perceived. Black-yellow, big-small, far-near, cold-hot. We perceive ourselves as separate from others and all objects appear to be separate entities. We can no longer perceive that underlying unified field or bond that links the manifested universe to the divine creator, because as mentioned before the manifest universe is an emanation of God himself. By recognizing the different colors, sounds, textures, tastes and smells the innocent child begins his sensual experiences and develops the ego-mind.

By transcending the ego-mind we re-connect to the universal field of energy, and remember that we are one with all of creation and the divine creator. All mystics, yogis and saints were in this level of consciousness. They see God in everything and everybody. As Jesus said the "Father and I are One". This reconnection or bond is what the word yoga means. The realization (the actual experience) that "I AM" an extension of all that exist, and not "I AM" the ego self, is the key to unlimited power.

It is said that our senses can either be used to liberate us from the world of limitations, or bind us to the world and its attachments. This will introduce an important concept in yoga; control of the senses. The yogi uses his senses to elevate his soul. This is the proper use of the senses.

We are all born as children of God this is why it is said that "in order to enter the kingdom of God one must become childlike". And truly one who has achieved yoga behaves much like an innocent child.

It is important to note that the freedom of choice is with us as human beings, and we can choose to do good or bad. We can choose to delve in the spiritual and speed up our spiritual progress or continue selfishly in pleasing the ego-self. Accumulation of material goods brings more worry and stress, and more attachment is connected to it, ultimately no true happiness comes from material gain, which is temporary like a fleeting shadow.

Yogis in India practice extreme detachment from the world by completely renouncing all their belongings and live in seclusion. In these modern days of course we find a lot of yogis who are householders, and have jobs. It is even more difficult to practice detachment while still in society, but never the less it is possible to live with detachment from worldly things. We must adopt the attitude of practicing this concept. All things in the physical universe are bound by change, decay and death. Knowing this, we don't accumulate material goods, we see our spouse, children and parents as the undying soul and we can accept the fact that they too will shed their bodies and are born into the realm of spirit, therefore though difficult it may be, no attachment should be developed towards them.

The other concept that we are going to discuss next is *Karma*. This word means both action, and reaction. Whatever choices we make in our dealing with others has a direct influence on our own selves. This is mainly because of our underlying unity as human beings. This concept of *karma* is explained in detail next.

About Karma

The process of yoga strengthens the karmic cycles. Karma means action and reaction, as in "what goes around comes around". What happens to us is a direct reaction to our own actions. You get back whatever you put out. It may take months, years, or a lifetime for the karma to come around, or it maybe almost instantaneous.

As yoga practitioners we should develop an attitude of non-violence and harmlessness. Specially if we live and work in the society, we can't afford the set backs we receive by producing bad Karma

Traditionally it is said that the blessings of a realized master is most necessary. The *guru* can help ease some of the negative past karmas. There are also some powerful yogic techniques that can clear past karmas.

It should be mentioned that both karma and attachments are causes of re-incarnation. When the soul is heavy with unfulfilled desires, attachments or bad karma, it will be forced to re-manifest in the physical realm to work out such issues. Since in Yoga we seek liberation from the limitation of the physical universe, and yearn to re-connect to the divine, we must be certain to let go of attachments, desires and karma.

Religion or Yoga?

Let me make it clear that yoga is not in contradiction to any religion. It will actually enhances your own religious convictions. In fact as we go through the process known as Yoga we recognize the greatness of the religion founders, and realize their courage and miraculous works better than their very followers.

World's great religions and their founders give humanity guidelines to help masses gain knowledge of the divine will. These religion founders are born to carry a specific mission for a specific time period. By following their teachings man receives salvation. Krishna, Noah, Abraham, Moses, Jesus are some of these great teachers who bring humanity social and moral laws and guide us to righteousness and nearness to the divine creator. Unfortunately religion has become from time to time the cause of disunity, hatred and war, which is absolutely not the intention of the great founders of these religions, but is caused by misunderstandings and misinterpretations.

Religion is to believe or to have faith. Humanity needs a place where they "belong", a group they can identify with, and laws to help the society function. As masses of people come together under the same belief they build new civilizations. Yoga on the other hand is not a mere belief but a scientific method of self-realization. The yogi will have a direct experience of the divine. He lives in a blissful state and enjoys "heaven" right here on earth. A truly accomplished yogi experiences his oneness with all of creation and his consciousness dissolves in the infinite, knowing that everything has come forth from the creator. He then experiences his or her oneness with God. Please remember this comes not as mere intellectualization but as a direct experience.

Following a religion may be an easier path, for by mere faith, and following some simple rules, you are promised to go to "heaven". This is why yoga seems less appealing to most people, because it requires the practitioner to follow a strict discipline, and to isolate to some degree and spend time in silent meditation, the yogi needs to be courageous and rely completely on God and trust that he will provide. But the fruits are worth the sacrifice, for as mentioned earlier the yogi actually gets the experience of the union and heaven right here on earth.

If you follow any religion you can still be a yoga practitioner. The yogi is a mystic. Going beyond the normal ritual of being a religious person, he has tapped into the very source of where these religious concepts have sprung forth. He or she may pick up any book such as the Bible or the Qhoran and fully comprehend the meaning or the wisdom behind the text. As the yogi reaches the higher levels of consciousness through the practice of yoga, all knowledge is revealed to him intuitively.

On the other hand if you have difficulty following an organized religion then be a yogi. Yoga is very universal and the truth becomes your own experience, not something someone imposes upon you. Yoga is all encompassing and all-inclusive, and does not discriminate. So whether you follow a religion or if you don't, you will benefit from the practice of Yoga. Just open your mind and don't be limited by your pre-conceptions, and enjoy the journey of unlocking the mysteries of the universe. Not just the physical universe but of all the spiritual universes. Also know that everyone is born with the potential psychic and paranormal abilities. These talents and abilities are developed and heightened through the practice of yoga, a luxury that you don't get by simply following a religion. It's important to note that gaining psychic powers should not be the goal. These so called powers (siddhis) are merely by-products of Yoga, and if misused for selfish gain or for harming others, will definitely destroy the practitioner.

Remember the process of yoga strengthens the karmic cycles. This is why one should keep the sight set on the highest goal, and avoid abusing, or showing off these psychic powers.

The Quest

Before we go any further let's recap some of the concepts we have examined so far so that we can proceed with a clear understanding of the process we are undertaking.

Since the ancient times, Man has always been fascinated with the natural Phenomena, and since his understanding of these phenomena was limited he attributed them to some powerful force and called it God. As the result of this he worshiped the Sun God, or the God of Thunder and lightning, the wind God, or the Fire God. This can be seen clearly in the Hindu religion, which is the oldest known faith on this planet, and these Gods are still honored today. Through ritual and sacrifice to these Gods of nature, man has tried to please them and win their blessing. Therefore formulated effective rituals to accomplish this.

If there is a drought, man prayed to the rain God or performed the rain dance, or if he was frightened by the storm, he prayed to the Gods of storm to spare him.

As man began to understand these occurrences as natural phenomena his search for God deepened.

His attention was soon turned onto himself. As he began to recognize himself as the greatest wonder of all, he began asking questions such as, who am I, what makes my heart beat? What makes it possible to breathe even when I sleep? Who is witnessing the dreams if my body is lying here with my senses shot down? And most importantly what happens when I die? These are questions we ask even today and these are the main driving force behind pursuit of mysticism and spirituality. The yogis were the first humans to speak of the existence of the soul, the true self.

This is where Mystics and Yogis separated from traditional religion of worship through ritual, and turned their attention from outside phenomenon to inner-self.

This process of going within to find the answers is known as meditation. Through meditation the ancient Yogis realized their true essence, which is called *Atman* or the Soul. "… And God created man in his own image". A popular verse which contains a profound truth. We know that God is not material it is spirit, so man is in his "image", and essentially a spiritual being or an "Angel".

All knowledge is known to the soul or *Purusha*, but his limitation as a physical being keeps him from accessing this knowledge. What is known as bondage is man's ignorance of his true self. Hypnotized by the play of nature (*maya*) he is seeking happiness in the material world forgetting that he is the all knowing immortal bliss. The process of emancipation (*vairagya*) or salvation is the journey of recognizing the true self within.

Therefore the mystics adapted special techniques by which they could transcend nature and arrive at their true self, *Atman*. These techniques known as the discipline of yoga helps transcend our limitations and gain access to all knowledge, not intellectually but through direct experience. One who has achieved yoga is no longer a simple man but a genius, saint or a truly God like individual.

And so the Journey began. As the ancient sages sought solitude and quiet for meditation, they journeyed into the forests and the mountains, fasting for days on end, denying themselves the luxuries of material life and resolved to find that spiritual treasure, immortality. It is interesting to note that the Buddha was fascinated by the yogis and had the same resolve. Jesus, Mohammad, Moses and other great teachers also spent time in the solitude of deserts, caves and mountains in fasting and solitude, much like the ancient yogis did. While in deep meditation they reached the highest levels of consciousness *samadhi*, and the truths that were revealed to them were passed down from the teacher to the disciple for thousands of years. This knowledge is sacred science of Yoga and *Vedanta*.

So to reach *samadhi* where the blissful ecstasy is experienced, we will have to follow certain guidelines that has been passed down for many millennia. This knowledge was compiled by sage Patanjali Maharaj in about 300 B.C. and is known as *Ashtang Yog* or the eight-fold path of Yoga. These guidelines are certain disciplines that we have to incorporate in our daily lives in order to reach the goal. Please remember that though we strive for perfection, we are most likely to fall short. Accepting this fact, we stay focused on the goal and will not allow small set backs discourage us. After all it is the journey that makes all the difference, and as long as we are making an effort, we are getting results.

What we are going to find here is an exact science of reaching the goal of self-realization. And without discipline and some sacrifice you are not going to get there. As we begin our journey of self exploration and self-realization, remember to honor the ancient Yogis who gave us this science, and with utmost respect bow at their feet, so that they may bless you with the inner mysteries of Yoga.

If you laugh at this or have too much pride to pay this respect you are not ready for the spiritual path. It is by loosing the ego-self completely that one can find the true self.

Faith in the divine and courage are of absolute necessity. Yoga is not for the weak or coward. It is the path of strength and courage. In the ancient days only kings and warriors who sought immortality used to take up this path. So if you are ready to experience the ecstasy of the divine and drink of the nectar of immortality, then step into the mystic realm of yoga.

CHAPTER TWO

Four Paths Of Yoga

There are four general paths to achieving yoga, that unitive state. No path is better than the other. Each path is suitable to certain type of individual's personality.

1-Karma Yoga: (yoga of action) This form of yoga is best for people with an outgoing nature. The practitioner is performing works without expectation of reward. Offering the fruits of action to the divine. Many of popular saints are of this type. They selflessly dedicate their life for the benefit of humanity.

2-Bhakti Yoga: (yoga of devotion) People of an emotional nature practice this form. By singing praises of the divine, praying and repetition of a mantra, the devotee merges with the divine. Singing praises of the Lord and loosing oneself in the devotion to God is Bhakti yoga.

3-Jnana Yoga: pronounced Gyana (yoga of knowledge). This path is almost like philosophy or intellectualization. It requires constant inquiry to one's own nature; by eventually transcending the physical body, the mind and the ego, the yogi will ultimately delves into his divine essence. The practitioner is heavily engaged in the study of the sacred texts and study of mysticism and different layers and levels of consciousness.

4-Raja Yoga: (the royal path). In this book when I speak of yoga I am referring to this path of yoga. The royal path is a scientific method of controlling and channeling the physical and mental energy and turning it into spiritual energy. Practice of yoga postures (Hatha yoga), breathing techniques (Pranayama) and silent meditation make up an important part of this path.

It is important to combine these paths, although the focus mybe to follow one of them as the main path. Raja yogi will benefit most for example, if his practice is mixed with some devotion towards the divine (Bhakti yoga), a little bit of inquiry to his own true nature (Jnana yoga), and a little bit of self sacrifice for the benefit of others (Karma yoga).

The purpose of this book is to examine exactly how this discipline called Raja Yoga can bring us closer to the goal. This is truly a science, because specific methods are used to take us from tangible results such as better physical, mental and emotional health to intangible results or the spiritual experiences.

Perhaps it is better to first discuss what yoga "is not". Although the word Yoga is a household word in the west, it is misunderstood by many. In the second half of the twentieth century the west became obsessed with Yoga and the health benefits of yoga postures. This "Exercise" aspect of Yoga is only a small segment of the discipline. The body is the temple of the soul, it is the vehicle our soul uses to go through this human experience, so keeping the body healthy and clean is an important aspect of spiritual growth. Therefore the yogis devised specific techniques known as Hatha Yoga to accomplish this. I am very hesitant to call those techniques a form of "Exercise", because aside from a few exercises that involves movement, hatha yoga focuses on specific "postures". These postures not only stretch and strengthen the muscles and the joints but also help us learn about stillness. A yogi may hold a specific posture for several hours looking almost like a statue. This physical stillness is the prelude to the stillness of the mind that we exercise in meditation. In a truly authentic form of hatha yoga, the postures are in fact a form of meditation and are not like aerobics exercises. Also a truly authentic form of Hatha Yoga would include the proper breathing techniques, and these three aspects—postures, breathing, and meditation are practiced simultaneously as well as separately.

With Yoga as a form of franchise, most Yoga Business establishments ignore or refuse to teach the authentic Yoga. There are commercial yoga studios who claim to be authentic, reading this book will help you decide whether or not they truly are so.

There are eight aspects that make up the discipline known as Raja yoga. By incorporating these aspects in our daily life we begin the practice of Yoga. These disciplines and practices are explained in the next segment.

To recap what we've studied so far as it relates to Raja Yoga, let's briefly go over the information given in the previous chapter. The word yoga means joining, union and bringing together. The goal is to achieve the unitive state of consciousness. Yoga is the process of bringing together and joining the individual's consciousness with the divine consciousness. For one who has truly experienced this unity, all things become possible. This duality or separation of the individual and the divine only exist due to ignorance. The ignorance is to believe that the individual is separate from the divine. This separation really does not exist, but man hypnotized by the play of maya has forgotten his true essence, and therefore lives in limitation. All the negative and painful experiences are due to this separation, but the consciousness of the one who has achieved yoga is always full of bliss, happiness and fulfillment. There are generally four types of Yoga. Other types of yoga fall within one or more of these main categories. The yogi is in constant awareness of the presence of the divine.

Raja Yoga The Eightfold Path

The science and discipline of yoga was compiled by a Sage known as *Patanjali Maharishi* about 2400 years ago. Many consider him a re-incarnation of *Vishnu* who appeared on earth to teach religion, medicine (*Ayurveda*) and Sanskrit grammar. He is the central figure and authority on these subjects. He explains the discipline of Yoga in his famous book *Yoga Sutras*. There are many translations and commentaries on the sutras, which you may choose to study. It is not my intention to produce another such book. I like to examine the concepts and explain them in a simple everyday language with the modern yogi in mind. These eight concepts are often practiced concurrently as well as in progression, as steps to *Samadhi*. Let us quickly examine these concepts.

1-Yamas: (restraints). The moral conduct, which consist of;
  a) Non-Violence
  b) Truthfulness
  c) Non-stealing
  d) Chastity
  e) Non-possessiveness

2-Niyamas: (observances) practice of which keeps the mind focused on the goal, and consist of;

a) Cleanliness

b) Contentment

c) Austerity

d) Study of the sacred texts

e) Surrender to, and awareness of the presence of God

3-Asanas: (yoga Postures)

4-Pranayamas: (regulation of breath)

5-Pratyahara: (drawing the awareness within) the stage of preparation for:

6-Dharana: (Concentration), which in turn will turn to:

7-Dhyana: (meditation), which will lead to:

8-Samadhi: (the state of super-consciousness). Here the yogi experiences enlightenment, ecstasy or Nirvana.

Let's take a closer look at these concepts. Everything here except *dhyana* and *samadhi* requires action; Things we do or practice, and remember as long as we make an honest effort to practice them we keep getting better at it. *Dhyana* just happens, and *samadhi* is the results we receive from our practice. The first two aspects are most important. *Yamas & Niyamas* are the daily moral conduct. The dos and don'ts. Without *yamas* and *niyamas* we don't have a strong foundation and are on shaky grounds. No matter how much you practice yoga postures or meditation you are not going to progress in the spiritual path, unless you are well established in the *yamas* and *niyamas*. Let's incorporate these principles into our lives immediately. These

moral conducts should eventually become a part of the charac-
ter, so the light of the spirit can shine forth.

1-Yamas

a) Non-Violence: basically means not causing any injury to any
living being. Non-violence must be practiced in thought, words
and action. If we constantly think about injuring someone
eventually this thought will lead to action. By stopping ourselves as soon as the thought of injury comes to mind, we learn
to control our actions. There are people who have caused us
harm and we seem to hold resentments against them. Write
down the names of people, places or things that make you
angry. Ask yourself why am I angry with this person? Now ask
yourself honestly how did I contribute to this resentment? Most
of the time we are angry because people did not act according to
our "expectations". It is our "Ego" that is keeping us in this
resentment. By harboring resentments we harm ourselves not
the person we are angry at. By lowering our expectations we
humbly accept the person or situation as it is and let go of our
anger. There are cases where we have honestly been a victim of
someone else's violence in this case we should pray for these
individuals and regard them as sick people who need healing.
By forgiving them we become much stronger spiritually.
Remember the spiritual principle Known as *karma*. This is
much like the law of physics, which states, "For every action,
there is an equal, opposite reaction". Our spiritual concept of

karma is similarly explained as "Do unto others as they may do unto you", or "what goes around, comes around". So every time one cause injury to others, or wishes another bad luck, that negative energy will come back to him, Even if the other person was at fault to begin with. It is not important what someone does to you, but what you do to others that affect you.

An important aspect of the practice of non-injury is eating vegetarian food. When we eat meat we contribute to the violent act of killing." Thou shall not kill" does not mention "except for food". While an animal is being slaughtered, it is going through tremendous levels of fear. This fear will remain in its body at the cellular level in the form of stored energy. Consuming this meat will make you agitated, angry and fearful. Science will soon discover many incurable diseases are contributed to consuming animal flesh. The meat industry often uses inhumane treatment and by feeding or injecting animals with hormones and other chemicals greedily attempts at producing bigger profits.

Some cultures have relied on hunting for survival, Such as Eskimos who had no way of cultivating vegetables. These cultures usually honored the kill and consumed the food only after proper ceremonies were performed.

Today's technology allows even Eskimos to receive fresh fruits and vegetables, so there is no excuse about why we, as an advanced species should not become vegetarians. History

reveals that human civilization began when man learnt to culti-
vate and engaged in agriculture.

Practice of this concept is difficult, although it is the sacrifice
we have to make for our spiritual growth. Conversion to vegetarianism should be done slowly and systematically. It may take
years to make a complete transition to vegetarianism.

Don't become a fanatic about being a vegetarian. Many meat
eaters who quit eating meat get the attitude of holier than thou.
This is pride and ego that should be combated at all cost.

We should avoid watching movies that promotes violence in
any form, or commercial ads that tempt us to eat meat. These
commercials are made after consulting psychologists to ensure
its effectiveness. These ads make the food appear very appetiz-
ing. Violent movies will agitate your mind.

Fresh fruits and vegetables provide all vitamins and proteins
the body needs. It is a fallacy to believe that we cannot live a
healthy life without meat in our daily diet.

Satvic or pure foods are most beneficial. This is first hand
food that grows on earth. Eating meat is second hand food, for
you are consuming an animal, which has in turn taken the first
hand food.

Fresh fruits, vegetables, legumes, organic milk and other
organic dairy products (free from Hormones and harsh chemicals) are considered satvic items.

b) Truthfulness: The most important aspect of truthfulness
is self-honesty. One must be willing to admit to ones own faults

and shortcomings. This is the stepping—stone towards progress in the spiritual path. Telling a lie or big talk should be avoided completely. I have not heard of a holy man or saint who had the habit of lying, or bragging. According to the *Yoga Sutras*, the person who always tells the truth gains such a power as to whatever he or she says will come true. For example he/she may say it is going to rain today, even if there is no cloud or anticipation of rain, suddenly clouds appear and it begins to rain. This is the power of speaking the truth always.

It is better to remain silent than to tell a lie. It is easy to make a habit of lying, and should be avoided.

c) **Non-stealing:** It is clear that when one takes something that does not belong to him, he is causing an injury to someone, which creates bad *karma*. There is no chance of spiritual growth when one engages in this unspiritual act. This act is also habit forming and I've heard that people do this act seemingly without reason.

d) Chastity:

As explained in the original scriptures, one of the yamas or observances is *Brahmacharya* or celibacy, which has a lot do with what we are trying to accomplish. If you are serious about yoga, you should first be firmly established in celibacy. We turn sexual energy into *Ojas Shakti* or spiritual energy. This is the ultimate goal, but remember even a householder can become a great yogi. This concept calls for bringing our senses under control. Many of the married yogis find it necessary to limit their sexual activity. Make sure your partner understands what you are trying to do and is supportive. Don't break your relationship because of this. Remember you have already made a commitment to be in a relationship and it is your duty to be there for your partner. It's best if you both are on the same path, but many people also grow apart which maybe inevitable. Be very cautious to not harm your relationship, because you are forcing your partner to comply with your new—found principle.

In some other forms of yoga discipline, the actual sexual union is used to produce heightened levels of spiritual ecstasy. This branch of yoga should be practiced with the proper guru and again teaching this may have turned into a business venture by some people, who are writing books about *Kama Sutras*. Be very careful.

For many, moderation is the key. This is not about sexual suppression it's about control. Remember we are human, as long as we make an effort we are making progress. It is important that we bring the senses under control. This is the process of eliminating the ego-self.

It is clearly explained in ancient text of yoga philosophy, and perhaps for the first time ever, how we respond to our surroundings and how the ego-self is produced. The five instruments of the senses which are, eyes, ears, nose, tongue and skin, provide information from the environment in the form of *Pancha Indryias*, seeing, hearing, smell, taste and touch respectively. This information is perceived by the mind (*mana*), then the intellect (*bodhi*) will process the information, and gives rise to ego (*ahamkara*). This is how we interpret the world around us as divided objects. There is the "I" and "This". We perceive ourselves as a separate entity from the rest of the universe, and all objects separated by color, texture, smell, size and so forth. The ego mind is what separates and divides everything. A new born baby who has not yet learned to use it's senses is free from ego, but as soon as that baby opens his eyes and begins to pay attention to sounds and the touch of the parents, it begins developing the ego-mind.

This ego-self is always seeking gratification from the outside world, and is sensual. Using the senses attempts to bring satisfaction and bliss. As mentioned earlier this will ultimately bind us to the material realm, and we cannot find satisfaction in the material world because it is constantly changing and decaying. The only thing that is eternal and real is the soul and to delve within to find this source of eternal happiness and bliss is to break away from the temporary worldly satisfaction. This is accomplished by keeping the senses under control. The yogi will establish a discriminative type of intellect, which will only accept the types of perceptions that leads to emancipation. In other words the yogi uses his senses only to elevate his soul.

These concepts are difficult to follow in a world where sex and violence is promoted constantly through the media. Some serious practitioners may quit watching T.V. altogether. Remember without some sacrifice we are not going to succeed in the spiritual path. If sex becomes troublesome spend more time in selfless service, so you don't have time to occupy your mind with sensual thoughts. Fellowship with people who are on a spiritual path (*satsang*) is a great support we all need.

e) Non-possessiveness: This concept in the original text is the principal of Renunciation. That is what yogis in India do even today. True renunciation is to live with complete detachment to the material world. As modern *yogis* and *yoginis*, we must pursue our calling in this world and continue to live within the society. I met one great saint from India, Shri Anandi Ma. She used to say "if one lives in the forest but his mind is in the city, he is not a *sanyasi*. One should be in the city and live with complete detachment to the material world; that's true renunciation". This is the concept of "being in the world, but not of the world". Too many possessions brings attachment and is a bar to spiritual growth. Unnecessary accumulation of wealth beyond ones needs is a sin. Giving to charity etc. is good *karma.*

Another aspect of non-possessiveness is non-attachment to people. Most marriages fall apart because the couples feel that they own each other. Unconditional love demands nothing in return.

2-Niyamas

Niyamas mean observances. Remember we should make a sincere effort at these concepts until they become engrained in our personality.

a) Cleanliness: This is both physical and mental cleanliness. We should keep the body clean at all times. Not just externally but also internally. There are yogic practices aimed at cleaning the body on the inside. This is known as *Pancha Kriyas.* Most importantly the nostrils, and the anus should be kept clean at all times. You should refer to a book that explains these kriyas in detail, or better yet, find a teacher who can show you how to properly do this. The other aspect is purity of thought. Negative thoughts are a bar against growth and success in any aspect of life

b) Contentment: To be content with every situation we are in, is a sign of total surrender to God's will. To be content is abundance. We must come to the realization that accumulation of materials does not produce happiness. In fact the opposite is true. The more "stuff" we have the more worries we carry. Longing for material goods brings attachment and that will make the process of emancipation much more difficult.

We usually dwell in the past regretting some decision we made, which cannot be reversed. We must learn from past mistakes and move on. Other times we worry about the future. Again projecting into the future and imagining how we will control situations that have not yet happened. This will keep us agitated and worried. To be content we must let go of the past and the future and be thankful for the here and now. As we learn to take each moment and live it fully we become more serene and focused, and make the right decisions, which will eventually lead to more contentment.

c) Austerity: Yogis in India go through some serious *tapas* or austerities. The yogi intentionally creates an unpleasant situation in order to achieve spiritual merit. One very famous form of *tapa* is fasting. Moses, Jesus and Mohammad prayed and fasted for days, in order to reach the highest levels of divine inspiration. Some yogis may balance on one leg or hold some difficult yoga posture for hours or days. During this period the yogi is engaged in deep meditation and will not quit until desired results are achieved. I personally like fasting for detoxification and as a form of austerity. There are many forms of fasting. The one that results in the highest spiritual reward is total abstinence from food and water. Native Americans, Muslims and Baha'is practice this type of fasting. I recommend that you get with someone to guide you every step of the way at least for the first day of fasting. You may fast for a day, three days or longer. By denying the body it's pleasures we bring the senses and desires under control. This is why some form of austerity is very beneficial.

d) Study of the sacred text: Doing this will keep us enthusiastic about our practice. It is important to study the knowledge that has been passed down through the ages, and understand the truths, which have already been revealed. Then we make these our own experiences, by practicing the concepts we have learned.

If you are interested in mysticism you must study the *Upanishads*. Also known as the Vedanta philosophy, the *Upanishads* are mystical utterances revealed to the ancient sages in meditation. There are numerous Upanishads and only ten of them are considered the main ones. Shri Eknath Easwaran does a good translation of the *Upanishads*, available through "Nilgiri Press". Another highly respected classic is the *Bahagavad Gita* which means the celestial song, or "The song of the Lord". This is also an Upanishad. The *Gita* is a segment of the epic story called *Mahabaharata*. In this beautiful poetic exposition, Lord Krishna reveals the different paths of yoga and instructs his devotee *Arjuna* in becoming a yogi. I recommend the Shri Easwaran translation again.

e) Surrender to God (awareness of divine presence): this is a very important concept. Without complete faith and trust in

God or the divine being we cannot tread the path of the spiritual. There are times that you feel you are not making any progress, or the trials in the path become overwhelming. You may become tempted and fall back. These are times that you need to have faith and surrender yourself to the divine and know that you are going to be alright. Placing yourself under the guidance and protection of the divine is an important aspect of the practice. The yogi eventually lives with the total awareness of the presence of the divine, and this is truly what is meant by total surrender to God.

3-Asana

Asanas are the famous yoga postures. In the west when you say "yoga" immediately people think of the postures. To some people this seems like a useless sport of twisting your body into a knot.

According to yoga, the body is the temple of the soul. We should keep the physical body clean and healthy. If we suffer from illnesses, we have little chance at spiritual growth. Asanas keep the body in top shape. The practice of the postures stretches and tones the muscles, and the joints. It has a positive effect on the blood circulation, boosts the immune system, and it stimulates the glands and the nervous system. More and more health professionals are recommending the practice of yoga postures. It is the cure for neck and back pain, digestive problems, irregular blood pressure, and many more health conditions.

When the postures are combined with proper breathing, it becomes helpful to conditions such as, anxiety, depression, fatigue, and bi-polar disorders. Aside from all the health benefits the practice of the Asanas eliminates tension and stiffness in the body, allowing the yogi to sit still for prolonged periods of meditation. I advise against practicing with books or videos that instruct yoga postures. The energy of a living guru is very beneficial. Also he or she can help you by correcting you. Understanding your limitations, a good teacher can help you build up slowly. Finding the right teacher is very important. Just because someone can perform the asanas with perfection, doesn't automatically make them a great yogi. On the other hand a great yogi may not be an expert in the performance of asanas.

A good teacher is compassionate and loving, and understands your limitations and will help you build up slowly. He or she should emphasize stillness, proper breathing and concentration as part of the practice of the asanas.

A teacher who demands extremely high fees, is in it for the money and is not practicing the *Yamas* and *Niyamas* which are the foundation of yoga and no matter how "famous" they maybe avoid them at all cost. Those who are chasing fame and money have completely missed the point and are not eligible to be yoga teachers.

You should feel calm and peaceful at the end of the session. If you want to sweat, take up aerobics. Yoga is not a "work out" and should not be approached as such. Best times to practice are early morning or in the evening. Don't practice in the middle of the day, if it's too hot. Never take a shower right after the *asanas*. If you do, you ground all the pranic energy you built during the practice, and this will defeat the whole purpose of practicing yoga postures. Wait at least four hours before you wash the body. I personally end the session with meditation. After all, the postures are performed to prepare you for meditation. That's another important point that modern practitioners have missed. Also know that when you do the Yoga postures you are practicing Hatha Yoga, There are different styles of hatha yoga usually named after the teacher such as Iyengar yoga, or Sivananda yoga, which are slight variations of Hatha Yoga.

4-Pranayama

Prana is the vital life force that is abundantly available throughout the universe. Scientists believe that the universe came into existence with a big bang. The Yogis have spoken of this for millennia. The static force behind the big bang is known as *Maha Kundalini*. As the universe began its expansion that primal energy turned dynamic and became the backbone of the physical universe. This dynamic energy is known as *Prana*. *Prana* continues to support life. Stars burn, planets turn and galaxies are formed and life exists because of *Prana*. We receive Prana mostly through the breath. *Prana* is not oxygen. Oxygen is a basic element that exists in the physical realm. Prana is spiritual energy and is our connection to the astral universe and beyond.

Prana is not gravity or magnetism. But these forces exist because of *prana*. We receive *prana* mostly through the breath. *Pranayama* is the science of bringing in prana to rejuvenate the cells in the body, to activate the energy centers or the *Chakras*, and to clear the astral passageways (*Nadis*) that carry prana to different parts of the astral body. It is used for healing oneself and others. At the physical level pranayamas are much like "breath-control", specific durations of inhalation, retention and exhalation.

Some pranayamas are considered to be the *kriyas*, which are used for both the internal cleaning of the body, and the clearing of the astral body. At the physical level fresh oxygen is sent to the blood stream, which is a way of detoxifying the body. Asthma, bronchitis and other breathing diseases are cured through the practice of *pranayama*.

There are many *pranayama* techniques and they should be studied and practiced under the supervision of a guru. After the practice of *Pranayama* you should feel rejuvenated, blissful and joyful.

Another aspect of *pranayama* is that it quiets the mind. The mind, the emotions and the breath are interconnected. For example if one is excited or frightened, his or her breath becomes very rapid. If shocked one may stop breathing momentarily and faint. On the other hand when we are relaxed or

sleeping our breathing is slowed down. The ancient yogis realized a long time ago that if we control the breath we can control
the mind, and therefore will be able to go into deep states of
meditation. These are the reasons why I emphasize proper
breathing even during the practice of asanas. A whole book
could be written on this subject alone but I have just told you
every thing in condense form. Later in this book we will learn to
practice some basic pranayams.

5-Pratyahara

Pratyahara means to draw our senses within. This is the process
of bringing our awareness from the outside environment to
within ourselves. With pratyahara we eventually shut down our
senses. Here we are starting the process of meditation. Many
important information may be revealed at this stage. when we
engage in pratyahara, we may suddenly remember an important
engagement that we had forgotten about. Write notes to self as
you work through this stage, so that after the meditation you
can attend to them. This also helps getting your mind off of it
now and not be worried.

As mentioned before our senses are constantly receiving
information from the environment, and this keeps our minds
occupied or agitated. The brain waves during normal state of
wakefulness are erratic. Moving at high frequency the mind is
constantly analyzing the information received by the instruments of the senses. Pratyahara is to let go of all that's going on

around us. We are bringing our awareness towards the point of concentration. Some meditation techniques begin by focusing on a single external object, such as a picture, or the flame of a candle. In this case pratyahara pertains to the process of letting go of all other objects in the surrounding and focusing on the point of concentration. It is the process of letting go.

6-Dharana

Daharana means concentration. To concentrate means to bring all our mental attention to a single point. The mind under normal functioning is constantly moving from one point to another. In other words the mind is undisciplined and likes to run off to different directions. In India they say the mind is like a monkey that likes to jump from one tree to another. Daharana is to bring the mind under control. It is the constant reminder of bringing the attention back to the point of concentration again and again. When you find yourself thinking about something else you should gently bring yourself back to the point of concentration. The mind is bound to wander off so just remembering to come back to the point of concentration is called dharana.

Concentration can be external or internal. Gazing at a candle, the picture of a saint or deity or listening to the river or the ocean is a form of concentration. It is best to choose something internal. Focusing on the breath, a *mantra,* or the *charkas* is a better alternative to external objects. Ultimately the practitioner looses all awareness of his environment and merges with the object of concentration and "falls" into meditation. This is very much like falling sleep which just happens. The effort is in dharana. Dhyana just happens as the result of concentration.

7-Dhyana

In dhyana (meditation) the effort for concentration has ceased, and the mind remains steadily at a single point. In other words the awareness is focused only on the object of meditation, and all concept of time and space has vanished. This is much like a continuous flow of liquid from one container to another. The meditator is lost in the "here and now" and the moment has expanded into eternity. In meditation though the practitioner is unaware of his physical body or it's environment, yet there is a great sense of wakefulness and awareness of the universe. Prolonged periods of meditation lead to the experience of samadhi.

8-Samadhi

Words cannot describe this state of consciousness. If I say "book", you think of several pages bound together, with covers to protect it, when I say "chair" you think of a four legged object with a back-rest used for sitting down, so the words represent something that you can visualize in your mind and the words help make sense of what I'm trying to say. The moment I try to explain the state of Samadhi I have limited the experience to something tangible in order for you to understand. So I have created a limitation of what this experience is. Much like trying to box it for you so you can see what it is. That is why it's difficult to describe the state of samadhi and it has to be "Experienced". All that can be said about samadhi is that it is the state of total peace and bliss. The practitioner's consciousness expands and the experience of oneness with all of creation is achieved. All knowledge is revealed as an "experience" of knowing, not just intellectual knowledge, but intuitional knowledge of the workings of the universe.

Generally there are two classifications of the experience of samadhi. The first one is called *Samprajnata* or *Sabija* meaning "with seed". In this state of samadhi the practitioner is absorbed in the object of concentration, but there is a sense of ego, or separation of the meditator and the object of meditation. Even though the two are merged as one the yogi is identifying himself as the object of meditation. The two have become one and yet they exist as an identity. In the second type called *Asamprajnata* or *Nirbija* samadhi meaning "seedless", there is an absence of ego, the self is lost completely and all that remains is "that" which is the object of meditation. This is the state of merging with the absolute, the state of the no-mind awareness. The soul is shining forth as an extension of the creator who has dreamed this creation.

The state of samadhi is reached in meditation, and when the meditation ends the yogi returns to normal, everyday consciousness. With continued practice the yogi reaches the state of consciousness known as *Nirvakalpa Samadhi*. The Buddhist concept of Nirvana is derived from this very word. In this state the yogi is always in the state of samadhi even while he walks or talks. All saints are usually in this state of consciousness. The separation of "I" and "thou" is vanished and total dissolution with the divine has taken place.

A yogi is capable of performing miracles and super-natural works such as healing with a mere glance or touch, appearing and disappearing, levitating or becoming heavy as a mountain. Walking on water, staying under water for days, or going without food or water for long periods of time. Such saints have appeared in India from time to time, and still exist though it's hard to find them in the cities. These super-natural powers are known as *Siddhis*. There are eight major and several minor siddhis that can be achieved with the practice of yoga. These *siddhis* are just by-product of yoga and should never become the goal. There are those who perform some miracles to gain fame or money. The scriptures warn us against such things. Our sights should be set on the goal, which is the direct experience of the divine. To the true yogi these powers are obstacles on the path. Thinking that one has become a great yogi because they are able to perform miracles is a boost to the ego. One must overcome the ego completely in order to find the true self. *Karmic* law is felt powerfully at this stage. If the *siddhis* are misused, it can quickly lead to self-destruction. A true yogi will discard these powers and sees them as mere indication that their efforts are bearing fruit. Therefore more enthusiastically they continue their *sadhana*. One who has attained one or more of these *siddhis* is known as a *Siddha*. I remember experiencing one of the major siddhis as a child. But because I was a kid and very afraid of this phenomenon, I learnt to stop such experiences whenever they occurred. The *siddhis* can be used to help other people on their spiritual path, and only then it is O.K to use them. Showing off, or trying to get some personal gain or satisfaction is extremely dangerous, and should be avoided completely.

About Hatha Yoga

The four aspects of *asanas* (postures), *Pranayama* (breathing), *pratyahara* (inner awareness), and *dharana* (concentration) together form what is known as Hatha Yoga.

Even though practice of hatha yoga is becoming more popular in the west, still a lot of people don't understand this as a sub-division of Raja yoga, and think of it as a form of fitness exercise. The most devastating thing I've come to find is that there are yoga competitions organized by so called authentic schools. How can one boost the ego about being a champion when the whole concept is to be rid of such attitudes? Yogis have been practicing yoga for many millennia and yet there are no competitions organized in India where it was originated.

They care nothing of the breathing techniques, inner awareness or concentration, and just pose this way and that way thinking they are going to become physically fit. A truly authentic form of hatha yoga should incorporate those four aspects as mentioned earlier. It's been my goal to introduce and teach this authentic form of yoga. In other words when practicing the postures one should combine it with proper breathing, draw the attention within, concentrating and holding still. We should learn physical stillness as we hold the postures, so that gradually we can translate this stillness to our mind during meditation.

There are many different styles of hatha yoga, Bikram, Ashtanga, Iyengar, or Sivananda yoga are some of the different styles of hatha yoga that are popular in the west. Most people think these are different "types" of yoga rather than different "styles" of hatha yoga.

The main focus in performing *asanas* should be to ultimately make the spine flexible and strong in preparation for the release of the *Kundalini Shakti*. Some styles of hatha yoga concentrate too much on strength building, and the main point is completely forgotten, which is making the spine flexible and strong. *Kundalini yoga* is a form of *Raja Yoga* (the Royal Path), and hatha yoga is it's sub division. *Kundalini* is that cosmic energy at the base of the spine. When awakened, this energy is directed up the spine towards the top of the head. The *kundalini shakti* will have to pierce through the five main *charkas* or centers of conscious energy located in the spinal column and two more within the brain. When this happens the yogi reaches the state of *samadhi*. This is an approach to enlightenment known as *Kundalini Yoga* and it should be practiced as a form of *Raja yoga*. In other words in *kundalini yoga* the foundation is *yamas* and *niyamas*, practice of *hatha yoga* will make the spine flexible and strong. Certain breathing techniques and meditations will activate and purify the *charkas* and helps awaken the *kundalini*

Shakti. So the path is *Raja Yoga,* with specific techniques geared towards the *kundalini* awakening.

Although there are specific methods of *pranayama,* and meditation that help accomplish the work of reaching enlightenment through *kundalini yoga,* it is believed that even if you practice *karma yoga* (yoga of action) or *bhakti yoga* (the yoga of devotion), the rise of *kundalini* is the cause of enlightenment. In other words even when practicing devotional chanting or *bhakti yoga,* we ultimately reach the state of *samadhi* because the *kundalini shakti* becomes activated during the chant.

To be successful one needs to begin by fully understanding the eightfold path of yoga as we have discussed so far, and put it into practice. Learning and practicing *asanas,* some basic breathing techniques and simple meditation as a daily routine is required before one attempts advanced, and powerful breathing techniques and intense meditations required to work with *kundalini.* This is why in the self-realization courses that I've been teaching, the first level is to fully understand and put into practice the contents of this book. The second level is the activation of the chakras and awakening of the *kundalini* which is beyond the scope of this book.

Nowadays anybody can become a certified yoga teacher. These new teachers may be very fit physically, because they have a background as a gymnast or dancer, and they can perform the advanced yoga postures with perfection. Yet the very same teachers may lack a good understanding of the yoga philosophy.

If the teacher is not practicing the *yamas* and *niyamas*, he or she is unfit to be a teacher even if they perform the *asanas* effort-lessly. On the other hand a great yogi may not be the best per-former of yoga postures. In fact perfection of asanas is the least important factor when we approach yoga as a tool for self-real-ization.

Sometimes there is great demand on the student to perform the postures with perfection right from the start. Proper align-ment and perfect posture comes with practice. A good teacher will understand the student's limitations and helps them build up slowly. Beware of the businessman.

About Meditation

Our consciousness is like a lake. Every time we have a thought, it's like throwing a rock at this lake. When the rock hits the water it creates a ripple on the surface of the lake. During the day and even during sleep the mind is very active. Our hundreds of thoughts and plans and desires are like hundreds of rocks thrown at this lake of consciousness, creating waves of distortion on the surface of the lake.

The process of meditation begins with concentration. Eliminating all scattered thoughts and focusing it on one point. Eventually this point is also dissolved, and our lake now comes to complete stillness, now we can see the bottom of the lake. In other words in meditation our mind has ceased it's fluctuations, so we can now delve deep within to find the true self. This is the whole purpose of yoga, to introduce us to the divine spark, the true self within. This is achieved by meditation. Daily practice is of utmost importance. Even if you sit for only five minutes, do it daily. Consistency is the key. Gradually you can increase the period of meditation. It is ideal to meditate for an hour without interruption. To reach the highest state of yoga three hours of non-stop meditation daily is required. With the daily practice of meditation, we achieve the final aspect, *samadhi* the state of super-conscious awareness, also known as nirvana. Of course if you meditate only a few minutes everyday you still enjoy the benefits of being centered, serene, and focused. You will perform whatever task with more efficiency. Once in samadhi you will remain effortlessly in prolonged periods of meditation.

Dharana (concentration), *dhyana* (meditation) and *samadhi* as a continuous process is called *Samyama*. One may perform *samyama* on the different *charkas*, a deity or an image or aspect of God. Whatever the approach, the results should be to attain the unitive state, where one's connection with the absolute or God is experienced.

Some people teach, "guided meditation". This is "suggestion" or "visualization" and should not be confused with yoga meditation, which demands letting go of fantasy and daydreaming and to focus on a single point.

So now we have a good understanding of this path called yoga, which ultimately lead us to emancipation. Living in the limitations of the three dimensional universe, and seeking satisfaction from something so temporary, is truly "bondage". Living with the awareness of the true self within which is limitless and immortal is known as emancipation or *kaivalya*. Yoga akes us from unreal to the real, from darkness to light and from bondage to emancipation.

The Five Afflictions

Man will remain in the darkness as long as he is suffering from the five afflictions. These five afflictions are the cause of man's sufferings. They are to be transcended by the process of yoga. Most of these concepts have already been explained, now let's take a look at these five afflictions.

1-Ignorance:

Mistaking the perishable for the permanent, pain for pleasure, that which is not the true-self for the immortal. Basically, attachment to the material world and hoping to find eternal happiness and satisfaction from the material, which is decaying and dying, is called ignorance. A true yogi views all his belongings as tools that aid him in the spiritual journey, and not wealth that is to be accumulated. Modern yogis should live with moderation and give to charity.

2-Egotism:

This concept was explained before. Here the individual is perceiving himself as a separate entity often in competition with other beings, and is constantly seeking satisfaction from it's surroundings. One's identification with one's gender, race, nationality, occupation, and even religion is an identification of the ego-self. The ego-self must be transcended in order to find the true-self.

Unlike the ego, the true self is in a state of bliss and total satisfaction already.

3-Attraction to pleasures (attachments):

This concept is also explained previously. Everything in the universe is constantly decaying and dying and there is no real happiness or permanent pleasure in this world. The more stuff we have the more worries we have and there is no happiness in the material world. Attraction to pleasures must be overcome. Pleasure is addictive and it becomes harder and harder to overcome it. To transcend this affliction the senses must be brought under control.

4-Hatred:

All afflictions are destroyed when the ego self has been transcended through yoga. Hatred cannot exist for one who has attained the unitive state.

5-Fear of Death:

Everyone including wise men have the fear of death. Only a true yogi, who has reached the highest levels of self-realization, truly recognizes that his physical body is not the true-self and that he is wearing it like clothing, in order to go through the physical experiences. The yogi is able to leave the body at will, much the same way as one removes his garment. This is one of the seven major *siddhis*. Pramahnsa Yogananda left his body at will and many yogis do this.

The practice of yoga will help the individual gain a better understanding of these afflictions and it helps to transcend them completely. Now there are eight obstacles that keep us from reaching the highest goal of transcending the afflictions and finding the true self. Let's take a look at these obstacles.

The Obstacles to Self Realization

The following are obstacles to spiritual advancement and must be overcome by daily practice of yoga. Specific methods are also incorporated to overcome the obstacles, for example the repetition of the mantra OM. We shall discuss this shortly. First let's get familiar with the obstacles.

1-Disease:

Disease is caused in three ways.

a) Self—inflicted: Caused by indulgence in pleasures of desire, lust and pride.

b) Chemical imbalance: when equilibrium of the five elements has ceased. Ayurveda is the science of restoring the balance and was developed and practiced by the yogis thousands of years ago. Using specific herbs and vegetables the equilibrium is restored.

c) Hereditary: genetic disease acquired at birth. This is part of the *karma* acquired in past life. As a child I used to wonder; "why some people are wealthy and some are born into poverty and why some people were born with certain diseases! Is it possible that God was favoring some over the others? How then can God be called kind and merciful?" Then I understood that these situations exist because of our own *karmas* in a past life. Remember that re-incarnation only takes place when there is too much attachment, unfulfilled desires, or when the soul is experiencing a lot of regret. The soul is so heavy that God out of his mercy may cause it to take physical form to work those karmas and desires. So based on our past life's karmas we are introduced to new challenges at re-birth.

We can overcome some of these conditions with the practice of yoga. In sever cases of disease practice of *raja yoga* may not be possible, but other forms of yoga such as *karma yoga*, or *bhakti yoga* may be more effective.

2-Mental Torpor or dullness:
It may be extremely difficult to achieve spiritual growth, if one suffers from major mental disorders. Some mentally challenged individuals may appear in a state of blissfulness, but in yoga true bliss is combined with extraordinary insight and wisdom, and those who are mentally challenged cannot reach that state. Another explanation of this condition is dullness, where the individual is just incapable of developing the necessary disciplines to reach enlightenment, and this maybe due to inexperience and lack of exposure to spiritual concepts in past lives.

3-Doubt:
There are times that one wonders if their efforts are paying off. They doubt that they are making progress on the spiritual

Path. Some may even doubt that spiritual growth is achievable. Faith in a supreme being is of extreme importance here. Continue your practice anyway. Don't stop! Inspiration comes from attending *satsang* or fellowship with like-minded people.

4-Indifference:

"Who cares about all this spirituality? Why should I waste my time with such practices", thinks one who is lost in the material world, and cares nothing of fulfilling his true purpose.

This way of thinking is of course a bar against pursuit of spirituality.

5-Laziness:

This is a very serious problem in the west. Every one wants that instant gratification. No body likes to work, and yoga is a discipline that requires daily practice. One should not lag on their practice especially on those days that motivation does not come easily.

6-Craving for Pleasure:

This is the nature of the beast. The more one pursues pleasure, the more one craves for more. Impressions left on the mind of the experience of pleasure is very strong and haunting. In yoga we bring our senses under control. Practice, practice, practice.

7-Delusion:

To have the false identity of the self is called delusion. Most people think, "I am a doctor" or an "engineer", or a "teacher". Some may even think "I am a great yogi", These are the identifications imposed upon the mind by the ego. The true self is not the ego.

8-Restlessness of the mind due to distraction:

The daily distractions are a bar against spiritual growth. This makes it impossible to concentrate. According to *Patanjali* the authority in Yoga philosophy, the whole purpose of yoga is to eliminate the movements and distortions of the mind and bring it into focus until the mind is completely merged with the object of concentration. Constant worry and pre-occupation with the material world is the main opposition to yoga.

Yoga postures and breathing also removes disease and depression. Control of the senses and keeping the faith will get you through the difficult times and temptations.

Continue the practice no matter what, and you will succeed. If you have a set back or get tempted don't feel guilty and don't beat yourself down. Forgive yourself and keep going. Most effectively these obstacles are removed by repetition and meditation on the sacred mantra OM.

What is OM

Sanskrit Language is the oldest known language. Its alphabet is based on sound vibrations. All of yoga philosophy is revealed in this language, and *mantras* are produced in Sanskrit.

A *mantra* is a sound formula that produces energy for a specific purpose. There are seed *mantras*, which are a single syllable, or compound *mantras* that could be a word or a sentence. These sound frequencies activate certain energy fields that could aid us in the spiritual path. *Mantras* are used to gain health, wealth, or most importantly used to gain spiritual growth. When *mantra* is used as the focal point during meditation, it is called a japa.

The *mantra* OM is the most universal of all sounds. All other *mantras* are made up of this universal *mantra*. In Sanskrit language the *mantra* OM (as shown on the cover of this book) is written such that it is made of three parts. The section that looks like the number 3, the part that looks like an O, and the segment that looks like a smiling face with a dot over it. The ancient texts that describe this *mantra* break it down to these three segments to explain its significance and meaning. So it would be appropriate to write this *mantra* as AUM. So when I give the explanation of its three parts or aspects, we can see it as A, U, and M.

AUM is the Sanskrit syllable, which basically represents GOD or the Absolute.

AUM is the most basic of sounds, it is said that the entire creation resonates to the sound of AUM. "In the beginning there was the word and the word was with God, and the word was God." That word is the sound of AUM. The yogis spoke about that big bang of creation thousands of years ago. This big bang is the explosive sound of AUM and as the universe expands, it continues to resonate to the sound of this *mantra*. I was blessed to experience this "sound" in meditation, just as the ancient yogis did thousands of years ego.

AUM represents all that is beyond past, present and future. It has always been and shall exist to eternity.

All words in every language are made up of this sound. Letter A is when the mouth is opened and the sound is produced, letter U is a modification made to the lips, and finally letter M when lips are closed to produce silence.

AUM also represents the divine trinity. Brahma the creator, Vishnu the Preserver or the Sustainer, and Shiva the destroyer or Renovator.

AUM represents the four states of Consciousness. A stands for the state in which the individual is awake. In this state the senses are receiving information from outside world, this information is analyzed by the mind and new impressions are formed.

U stands for Dreaming state, where the senses are shut down, and the individual is witnessing a world based on past experiences and present desires.

M stands for the Dreamless sleep. In this state the soul rests in it's own splendor but the individual is not aware of this. If he becomes aware of this state he is in the bliss of Brahma.

But AUM Cannot be divided therefore A-U-M together represents a fourth state of Consciousness known as *Turya*. This is the state of super-consciousness where the individual experiences the unitive state. May you attain it through the repetition and meditation on AUM.

Repetition of AUM with feeling will eliminate all afflictions, and removes all obstacles in the path of Self-realization. With it's resonating quality it will cleanse and open the *Chakras* the centers of conscious energy located along the spinal column and the *Nadis*, conduits that transfer cosmic energy or *prana* to all parts of the astral body, much like veins in the physical body, which distribute blood to throughout the physical body. It is most beneficial when OM is repeated out loud. But you can also whisper it or quietly in your mind for the same effects. All the yoga and mystical scriptures begin with AUM and end with,

AUM.... Shanti, shanti, shanti

CHAPTER THREE

Daily Sadhana

Yogis in India begin just before sunrise and bathe in the holy river of Ganga. This is always a good start, cleaning the body. If you perform internal cleaning or the *Kriyas* you should perform it before you begin your *Sadhana.* It is important to remember that you should never wash your body after the practices. Washing the body after the *sadhana* will also wash away all the *Shakti* you have been building through your practice. In other words all the spiritual energy built up within is grounded.

A clean body affects the spirit, because the physical and spiritual self is interconnected.

Next we sit down and recite an opening prayer. This should be such that you pay your respect to the ancient sages and the yogis, who have given us this science of self-realization. Traditionally The Guru Mantra is recited honoring God as the teacher.

"OM … Gurur Bramha, Gurur Vishnu, Gurur Devo Maheshvara, Gurur Sakshad Para Bramha Tasmei, Shri Guruve namaha."

In our English prayer the words are not that important as long as you express the general idea or say something like this:

"Salutations to the inner Guru, who brings infinite knowledge and ultimate bliss.

I bow down to the saints and sages. O divine protector, aid me in my efforts. Bring me closer to the height of thy sanctity.

Protect my teacher and I from all harm".

Then we begin the sequence of Asanas with the *Surya Namaskar* (sun salutation). This should be done while facing the rising sun. If you know the special mantra that draws energy from the sun for vitality and protection recite it before you begin the exercise. The sun salutation stretches all the major muscles, gets the heart pumping and warms up the body. Then continue with the rest of the yoga postures. There are of course standing, sitting, laying down and balancing poses. It's important to follow a routine that starts out with easy poses and builds to more difficult ones, rather than some random postures.

You should finally come to a cross-legged sitting position known as the lotus posture (*Padmasana*). Now you will perform any special *pranayamas* that was recommended to you by your teacher. The pranayamas further charges you with the *Prana Shakti*, and clarifies the blood by sending fresh oxygen to it, clears the respiratory tract and most importantly, it will quite your mind and prepares you for meditation.

The process of meditation begins with *dharana*, concentration and will eventually lead to *samadhi*. If you are beginner start with five or ten minutes of meditation and eventually increase this period till you can comfortably sit still and meditate for at least half an hour. On your days off when you have more time you should try to extend your meditation, and meditate longer than normal. But even five minutes of meditation is extremely beneficial, if practiced as a routine.

Finish with the final relaxation, at which time you relax every part of the body, then get up for the closing prayer. Again the wording is not that important as long as you express the general idea. Thank the divine for having had the opportunity to do your spiritual practices. Say something like this:

"I thank the creator, the great spirit, God, for helping me practice yoga today, so that I may have a healthy body, healthy mind, and a healthy spirit, so that I may know the Self better. I am grateful
Om ..., Shanti, Shanti, Shanti"

In Sanskrit I recite the following closing prayer.
"OM ... Ananda Mananda karapasannam, Gyana Swarupam Nejabo Darupam. Yogendra midiyam, Bahavarogya vaidyam. Shrimat Gurum Nityam Maham Bhajami.
Om ... Shanti,Shanti, Shanti"

It's a good idea to pray for your friends, family, the world of humanity, planet earth, peace on earth or anything or anybody else as well. Never pray just for yourself. Remember the sick friend, innocent people dying at war, hungry children all over the world or the endangered species vanishing because of man's greed. The more enlightened you become, the more you feel and understand such sufferings. Your consciousness is no longer limited to selfish wants and desires, and you will want to get up and go out to make a difference.

As you go about your business during the day, remember to practice the *yamas* and the *niyamas*, the moral conduct we studied earlier.

Through your new found serenity your interaction with the world around you changes and other people's short comings and ignorance will not bother you as much. You see everything in a new light, and are able to forgive and forget a lot easier.

Even if you feel you are an expert at the performance of *asanas*, you should still continue attending yoga classes regularly. Being in the atmosphere of a class with the energy of a good teacher is very beneficial. Find like-minded people or those who use the same meditation technique and meditate with a group at least once a week.

Give to charity and engage in selfless service. Every chance you get, go out of the city to where you are closer to nature and perform your *sadhana* there. Take sometime to ponder upon questions such as who am I? Why am I here in this body? And

ask God for guidance. Some devotional chanting is also beneficial. Enjoy the journey and don't expect quick and profound
results from your practices.

Attend *satsang* to listen to a lecture or an explanation of yoga
philosophy from a guru. Study the *Bahagavad-gita, Upanishads*
or other yoga related scripture or other spiritual books.

In the evening spend a few minutes to ponder upon your day.
If you have harmed anyone and if you owe someone an apology
do it promptly.

Keep the faith and don't give up. Tell your friends how good
you feel about being a yoga practitioner and inspire them to get
on the path. May God's blessing be upon you every step of the
way.

Asanas Applied

It is not my intention to produce a book about yoga postures, and in fact I always tell people to refrain from practicing with videos, or books. It is imperative to begin your practices with a qualified guru, and when you have reached a level of confidence, that you feel comfortable doing the practices on your own, you can have some reference materials to help you along the way. It is easy to get injured if you are not careful, and where there is no one to help you. Books and videos are prepared using professionals, but the beginner who feels compelled to do those advanced postures may find himself in a lot of pain. Therefore I will just write about guidelines of proper practice to help you find the right teacher, and know to a degree if what they teach is truly authentic.

It is recommended to practice the *asanas* on a yoga mat, because it keeps you from slipping and falling. I don't believe in dependence on props but as a safety feature recommend the use of the yoga mat.

The word asana means "seat" or "sitting", and the sitting posture is the only one we need to master. Meaning we should be able to sit still for long periods of time to meditate. All the other

Asanas or postures were eventually developed to strengthen the body and to relieve tension and stress so that we can sit still and meditate. Another point that is most important is that aside from strengthening the muscles, and stress relief, the postures should be used to make the spine flexible and strong. Modern practitioners often ignore this. Even if you practice the postures strictly for health reasons, remember that with a flexible and strong spine, you will look and feel young and healthy. Generally you bend and arch the spine forwards, backwards, sideways and twist it in all directions, plus any combination of the bending and twisting.

Never practice on your own with a book or video. Especially in the beginning you need to have a teacher demonstrating and explaining the asanas, and of course correcting you if necessary. I don't want to make this book on yoga postures, so I will explain what's most essential. The "exercises" are movements from one pose to the next, and the "postures" are "held" in complete stillness.

It is important to understand that there are three segments in every posture: going into the pose, holding the posture, and coming out of it. After each posture we must return to relaxation pose or *savasan*. Doing so will allow the pranic energy to flow in the body, and you may feel this in the form of pulsations or energy movement. If no time is given for this, the exercise becomes too strenuous and the main objective is lost. Going into and coming out of the postures are always "synchronized" with a breath. You will breath into the pose and breath out of the pose. One should practice with a guru to learn the proper way, there is no specific rule to this but if the breathing is not done properly the practice maybe harmful rather than beneficial. In a general way raising the arms or legs is done with an inhalation, while lowering them is accompanied with exhalation. Exhale when crunching the abdomen, unless you are raising your legs. There is always exceptions to these rules. While you hold the posture, close your eyes and bring your awareness within yourself. You become physically still like a statue, but you will continue with the peaceful abdominal breathing. As you breathe peacefully in the pose you should focus on the breath. Observe the incoming and outgoing breath. Most preferably you will be repeating a *mantra*. There are a few exceptions when you hold the breath as you hold the posture. *Pratyahara* or that inner awareness is also combined as you practice the postures. For this you will keep your eyes closed as you hold the posture. Most modern studios advise against closing the eyes, because you may loose your balance and fall. This poses a threat to their "business", since you may want to hold them responsible for your injury. If you have trouble keeping your balance, keep your eyes open, but as you get better at it, do it with eyes closed. So you should have a good picture of how *hatha yoga* is practiced. It is really a combination of *Asanas*, *pranayamas*, and meditation. You practice with your eyes closed, you will breathe into, and out of the pose, and while you hold the posture you are meditating by focusing on the breath and or a *mantra*.

Before the practice of *asanas* we begin with an exercise to warm up. This exercise is called *Surya Namaskar*, or "sun salutation". Honoring the "Sun God" is both scientific and spiritual. Life cannot exist without the sun, so respecting the sun should be a natural part of our existence. The yogis recite specific *mantras* to draw energy from the sun, for vitality, strength, and protection. *Surya Namaskar* will stretch and tone all the major muscles, gets the heart rate up and warms up the body in preparation for the other postures. As a beginner if this exercise is all you do, you have done a lot. The sequence of postures in this exercise includes forward and backward bends; it strengthens and tones the major muscles. Remember to stay on the mat throughout the exercise. Move slowly and meditatively and breathe into the movement. You can do the postures in any order you like, postures in sitting position, standing position, lying on the back and laying on the stomach, but maintain a routine of the postures you perform in each category. Don't try to change your routine, don't try new postures everyday and don't practice random postures, follow a routine and stick to it, practice makes perfect and promotes discipline. The routine should begin with simple postures and exercises and build up to more difficult ones. Extremes should be avoided. I cannot emphasize the importance of a good teacher. Remember just because someone is flexible and can perform the postures with ease, doesn't qualify them to be a yoga teacher.

Pranayamas Applied

Once I decided to attend a yoga class, and I do this once in a while to see how others approach yoga. I called and told them it was my first time with them, that I would like a beginner's class. To my surprise the teacher had everyone doing advance pranayamas. Very scary, I thought because this was going to be too overwhelming for most people, and harmful to total beginners.

Please approach yoga slowly and gradually. Even the spiritual concepts should be established slowly and systematically, otherwise it becomes too overwhelming and discouraging. So let us take it slowly. In the previous chapter we discussed the benefits of *Pranayamas*, please refer back to that section and re-read for a refresher.

Pranayama is the single most important aspect of Yoga. The first thing we require when we are born, is the breath. You can go several days without food or water, but without air we die instantly. Although *pranayama* relates to breathing, it's main purpose is to bring in *prana* or the life force. This life force is spiritual energy not oxygen. Since we receive *prana* mostly through the breath, the techniques appear to be physical. The benefits are not only powerful spiritual experiences, but it also brings peace of mind, clarity and focus.

I will explain the foundation and the basics of *pranayamas* so that you can begin practicing it and receive the benefits of it. Practice the pranayamas in sitting position. You can use the simple sitting pose (*Sukasana*) or the half or full lotus (*Padmasan*).

Abdominal Breathing

Even though this is a very basic form of pranayama, but it is also the most important. You will do this type of breathing when you are practicing the asanas, also you will use it for meditation. In this technique you breathe very peacefully. As you inhale the abdomen rises. When you exhale the abdomen will go in. put your hand on your abdomen so you can get a feel for this. Inhale and exhale through the nose only. Your abdomen rises and falls subtly as you breath peacefully. Sustain the breath by controlling the amount of air coming in and going out. You can mentally count to three as you inhale and as you exhale. Inhaling through the nose mentally count 1 and, 2 and, 3 and, then exhale through the nose and extend it to the count of three, 1 and, 2 and, 3 and. You will immediately feel the benefits of this pranayama. If you just stay focused on the breath like this for a few minutes, you are actually meditating. The best meditation technique would be to eventually let go of the counting the numbers, and instead inhaling and exhaling the mantra OM. Extending the inhalation and exhalation for three seconds. We will discuss meditation in the next segment.

Deep Yogic Breathing

Inhale and exhale through the nose only. We are going to control the "amount" of air coming in and going out in order to "sustain" the breath. It should take five to ten seconds to fill up the longs to the top raising the chest profoundly. Then it should take from ten to twenty seconds to exhale. This extension of exhalation is accomplished by pushing the abdomen in towards the spine during the exhalation. As soon as you are finished inhaling begin the exhalation. Similarly as soon as you finish exhaling, begin the inhalation. There should be no pause in between. Do not hold your breath. Remember it takes practice to get comfortable with these breathing techniques. Practice makes perfect. A live teacher is most beneficial.

Just learning and practicing the two types of breathing I have described here you will be able to get a lot of benefits. You will use these *pranayamas* for meditation in the next section.

Grounding technique

Do the deep yogic breathing as described above. As you inhale for up to ten seconds visualize the positive spiritual energy is rising up the spine, from the base of the spine towards the third eye. On the exhalation which takes ten to twenty seconds visualize a chord attached to the tailbone on one end and connecting to the core of the earth on the other end, and as you exhale send all the negativity, anger and frustrations, down that chord to the core of the earth. Do this visualization with your deep breathing for about ten deep breaths, then allow yourself to relax gradually, and slowly and as you relax your breathing will automatically change to the peaceful abdominal breathing. Do this exercise at the beginning of your *sadhana* to get rid of negativity, or during the day when you feel frustrated.

Yoga Meditation applied

After you have practiced your postures and any advanced *pranayamas*, you are ready for meditation.

Let us incorporate the sacred Mantra OM. This mantra is very universal, is not tied to a deity and is not affiliated with a religion. But it is important to note that Hindus have used this mantra for thousands of years.

It is a good idea to do more prayers at this time, maybe just asking to be successful in your meditation. Sit in a simple pose (*Sukhasana*), or the lotus posture (*Padmasana*). It is important that you are comfortable. Keep the spine erect. Head should be in a straight line with the spine. Close your eyes and put your gaze at the point between the eyebrows (the third eye). To accomplish this with your eyelids closed roll your eyes up and in, as if you are looking at a point between the eyebrows. By so doing you will eventually open the "third eye" which is the seat of the soul, and the center for clairvoyance. As a beginner your eyes may hurt or you may experience a headache. To eliminate this discomfort, imagine the point between the eyebrows to be two or three inches away from your face in front of you. This will make it a mild, gentle gaze.

First begin with a few Deep breaths. (Refer to the previous section,Pranayamas applied). After ten deep breaths gradually allow yourself to relax until your breathing changes to the peaceful abdominal breathing.

Now as you do the abdominal breathing, establish a rhythmic pattern of inhaling and exhaling to the count of three. Focus on your breath. As you do the peaceful abdominal breathing, inhale … 1 Om, 2 Om, 3 Om, then exhale 1 Om, 2 Om, 3 Om,…. stay focused on this inhaling and exhaling to the count of three for about a minute or two. By this time you have established a steady, peaceful and rhythmic breathing pattern. You can now let go of the counting. Instead, inhale Om…. for three seconds, exhale Om … for three seconds. Now you are focused on the point of concentration.

Of course in the beginning your mind will wander. This is normal since the mind is undisciplined and likes to run off in different directions. You may remember an important engagement as you clear your mind, write this down so you don't forget to attend to it later and then let go of it and come back to inhaling and exhaling to the count of three. If your mind wanders off to something that's not important, learn to look at yourself as an observer and think such, "look at me I'm Thinking about something else again! Let's bring me back to the point of concentration". This way you are being non-critical of yourself. Remember, this is the first stage of meditation; bringing yourself back again and again to the point of concentration.

After a while with practice you will be able to stay focused on the *mantra*. As you learn to meditate and prolong the focus, one of two things can happen:

You become one with the object of meditation—in this case the *mantra* and this is why it's important that you understand what the mantra represents. Do the repetition of the mantra with feeling, as it represents something profound or sacred, so as you merge with the mantra you are becoming "one" with that divinity.

The other condition is that the point of concentration (the Mantra) dissolves and you enter the "no-mind" state of consciousness. In this state, the breath, the mantra and everything else has ceased to occupy your mind.

Now you are beginning to experience *samadhi*. I should say you are beginning to scratch the surface of experiencing the ultimate bliss, Nirvana, or super-conscious awareness. Don't get discouraged if you don't get to this stage right away, it may take several years of routine, daily practice to get there. But if it is the divine will, you will get the experience a lot sooner. Also if you get the experiences and you are achieving the results, don't become too excited and think that you are becoming a great yogi. That is the ego-mind fooling you again. Stay humble and keep practicing. The intuitive and psychic powers are heightened as you practice. Don't abuse these powers, it will become a setback in your progress.

Maintaining a daily routine with your practice is extremely important. On the days that you have more time, extend the Sadhana.

Finish the meditation with a few deep breaths and then a closing prayer. Now you are bringing yourself back to every day normal consciousness, so as you do the closing prayer, don't pray just for yourself. Pray for friends, family, the world of humanity, planet Earth, Peace on earth so as you bring yourself back you are reconnecting with the ultimate mission of bringing peace, harmony, and healing to those you encounter as you go about your business. You may choose to lye down in the relaxation pose for a few minutes, but after you get up slowly, you will feel very focused and energized.

Final words

I hope more people would become true yogis. As the inner transformation takes place, it reflects on the outside and a great change is felt all around. As the yogi reaches the state of enlightenment and realizes that the underlying all that exist is the divine love and experiences the unitive state, there is no longer "you and me" or "us and them", no "right and wrong" no "better or worse". The yogi will want to contribute to the world without any expectation of reward because he sees everyone as an extension of himself. A new form of global economy will emerge as more people recognize their true purpose and potential. As the divine inspiration flows, arts, crafts and sciences will take on a new dimension and the world will be transformed. As people of the world work together in co-operation rather than competition, our true potential as a species will reach new heights and as our unity is established world peace will become reality. The age of ignorance and darkness ends and a new era will dawn, where humanity will truly live as one. We will no longer abuse our resources and see this unique and beautiful planet as an extension of ourselves, a living entity. Plants, animals and humans will reach a perfect equilibrium. This is what is known as heaven on earth, and although most people are hoping and praying for the kingdom of God on earth, little will be accomplished unless we begin to take responsibility for our own selves, and resurrect the divine inspiration or the "Christ" within us.

May the divine light of love shine upon all the peoples of the world.

Om, Shanti, Shanti, Shanti....

Terminology

Ahamkara=The Ego-mind

Asana=Yoga Posture

Asamprajnata=literally means "Without seed". The no-mind consciousness.

Atman=Soul

Arjuna=Lord Krishna's prime devotee.

Brahma=the creative aspect of god. One aspect of the divine trinity. Brahma the creator, Vishnu the sustainer, and Shiva the destroyer or renovator.

Brahmacharya=Celibacy.

Bhagavad Gita=literally means "the song of the lord". A popular book that explains different forms of yoga.

Bodhi=intellectual mind.

Chakras=literally means wheel. energy centers. Centers of conscious energy.

Dhyana=meditation

Guru=A spiritual teacher. A master

Hatha Yoga=the practice of yoga postures, breathing techniques etc.

Kaivalia=liberation. Freedom from the limitations of the maya.

Kriyas=Cleansing techniques

Krishna=A manifestation of God on earth, re-incarnation of Vishnu

Kundalini=Cosmic energy, dormant at the base of the spine, activating this energy and directing it to the brain brings about enlightenment.

Kundalini Shakti=Kundalini Force or energy.

Kundalini Yoga=the practical techniques of awakening and controlling the Kundalini.

Mana=Mind. Analytical mind.

Maya=manifest universe. The illusion of individuality and separation.

Mahabharata=an epic story which is the backbone of modern Indian culture.

Mantra=A sound formula. By repetition of a mantra the mind is liberated. "man" means mind and "tra" means to liberate.

Nirbija=seedless. The state of "no mind" consciousness

Niyamas=the moral observances. The second "limb" of yoga philosophy.

Padmasana=The Lotus posture. Yoga sitting position used for meditation.

Pancha Kriyas=the five internal cleansing techniques.

Patanjali=A highly respected sage who lived around 300 B.C. He is considered to be a master of yoga philosophy. The author of the "yoga sutras".

Prana=the vital life force.

Prana Shakti=Pranic energy, used for healing others or ones own self.

Samprajnata=literally means "with seed". The seed is the object of meditation. A state of consciousness where the practitioner becomes one with the object of meditation.

Samyama=concentration, meditation and enlightenment as a continuum.

Satsang=a spiritual gathering, usually involves chanting, meditation and lecture by a guru.

Karma=the law of cause and effect.

Ojas Shakti=spiritual energy.

Purusha=the human Soul. The higher self.

Pancha Indryas=the five senses of seeing, hearing, smell, touch and taste.

Pratyahara=drawing the awareness within.

Rajasic=the state of excitement. Food that excite the passion. One of the three qualities of nature. The three states of nature are Satva, Raja and Tama.

Sabija=Same as Samprajnata. Literally means "With seed. The seed is the object of meditation. A state of consciousness where the practitioner becomes one with the object of meditation.

Sanyasi=one who belongs to the renounced order. A monk. One who lives without any attachments.

Samadhi=enlightenment. The state of Super-consciousness.

Sadhana=Spiritual practices

Satvic=Pure. State of purity. Pure foods. One of the three qualities of nature. The other two being Rajasic, and tamasic.

Siddhi=Psychic powers. Ability to perform miracles.

Shakti=Energy

Shiva=the king of yogis. One of the three aspects of the divine. Brahma the creator, Vishnu the sustainer, and Shiva the destroyer or renovator. Shiva destroys the lower or the animalistic nature and gives rise to the higher spiritual self. Usually shown sitting in meditation.

Surya=the sun, or the Sun-God

Surya Namaskar=Sun salutation. A hatha yoga routine that stretches the major muscles, speeds up the heart rate and warms up the body

Tapa=Austerities. Self inflicted hardship for the sake of spiritual growth. The control of the lower nature.

Upanishads=also known as the Vedanta philosophy. The mystical utterances revealed to the yogis during meditation.

Vairagya=non-attachment. Renunciation.

Vedanta=the end of the Vedas. The final chapter of the book of Vedas. Also see "Upanishads".

Vishnu=One of the three aspects of the divine. Brahma the creator, Vishnu the sustainer, and Shiva the destroyer or renovator. Vishnu re-incarnates whenever there is un-religion or chaos in the world. Some of his manifestations are Krishna, Rama, and Narayana.

Yamas=the observances. The famous moral conducts that is the first "limb" of the yoga philosophy.

Yogi=a practitioner of Yoga. One who has attained higher levels of consciousness through the practice of yoga.

Yogini=A female practitioner of yoga.

978-0-595-47854-5
0-595-47854-9